Table of Contents

Gastric bypass is a surgical procedure that can help people with obesity to lose weight and improve their health. It decreases the size of the stomach and changes the way the stomach and small intestine absorb food, making it easier to lose weight. This procedure is also called a Roux-en-Y gastric bypass.

Gastric bypass surgery is a metabolic and weight loss procedure. It's also known by the French term, "Roux-en-Y." The procedure works by modifying your digestive system so that you consume and absorb fewer calories. It modifies your stomach and also your small intestine.

Like other bariatric surgery operations, gastric bypass is recommended for people who have clinically severe obesity. It has been shown to help relieve a long list of obesity-related health conditions, including type 2 diabetes, hypertension, obstructive sleep apnea and GERD (chronic acid reflux).

If you are very obese and have other health problems, and have tried hard to lose weight by dieting and doing more exercise, your doctor might suggest gastric bypass surgery to help with weight loss.

Gastric bypass surgery is a very effective type of surgery for weight loss, but it is not for everyone. Discuss with your doctor which approach is best for you, and talk about what to expect.

Roux-en-Y Gastric Bypass (RYGB) — pronounced "roo-en-why" — is the most commonly performed weight-loss procedure in the United States. It has been in practice for more than 30 years and provides an excellent balance of weight loss and manageable side effects. The operation can be performed laparoscopically (small incisions to the abdomen) or robotically (computer-assisted surgery used to aid in surgical procedures).

A gastric bypass is where surgical staples are used to create a small pouch at the top of the stomach.

The pouch is then connected to your small intestine, missing out (bypassing) the rest of the stomach.

This means it takes less food to make you feel full and you'll absorb fewer calories from the food you eat.

GASTRIC BYPASS DIET RECIPES

BREAKFAST

1. Baked Ricotta Florentine

Prep Time: 10 Minutes

Cook Time: 15 Minutes

Servings: 4

Ingredients

- Olive oil spray extra virgin
- ¼ cup fresh spinach, chopped fine
- 2 tablespoon minced sun-dried tomatoes
- 8 oz. ricotta cheese full fat or part-skim
- ½ cup shredded mozzarella cheese
- 2 tablespoon grated Parmesan cheeese

Instructions

1. Preheat your oven to 350 degrees F.
2. Grease your ramekins with olive oil.
3. Spray a saute pan with olive oil and heat to medium heat.

4. Saute chopped spinach in the saute pan until wilted.

5. In a medium bowl mix together ricotta cheese, mozzarella, parmesan, spinach, sun-dried toamtoes.

6. Divide mixture evenly among greased ramekins.

7. Top each ramekin with additional shredded mozzarella.

8. Bake for 15-20 minutes until cheese is melted and slightly browned.

2. Turkey Bacon Burritos

Prep Time: 5 Minutes

Cook Time: 15 Minutes

Servings: 10

Ingredients

- 10 Slices turkey bacon, cut into 1/4-inch pieces
- 1/2 Cup green pepper, seeded and chopped
- 1/2 Cup onion, chopped
- 5 eggs
- 1/2 Cup skim milk
- 1/4 Teaspoon pepper
- 1 Cup reduced-fat Cheddar cheese, grated
- 10 8-inch flour tortillas
- As needed Salsa

Instructions

1. In large non-stick skillet, over medium heat, cook bacon, green pepper and onion 12 to 15 minutes or until bacon is lightly browned, stirring frequently. Regulate

heat to prevent sticking and burning; remove skillet from heat.

2. In small bowl combine eggs, milk and pepper. Pour egg mixture over bacon mixture. Return skillet to low heat for 2 to 3 minutes or until eggs are almost done; stirring frequently. Remove skillet from heat and stir in cheese.

3. Place 1/4 cup egg mixture on lower 1/3 of each tortilla. Roll tortilla and place in 9 X 13-inch microwave-safe dish; cover with plastic wrap. Cook in microwave oven at HIGH (100% power) 2 to 3 minutes or until burritos are hot.

4. To serve, drizzle salsa over burrito.

3. Better Casserole

Prep Time: 20 Minutes

Cook Time: 35 Minutes

Servings: 18

Ingredients

- 8 ounces (1 recipe) low-sodium breakfast sausage
- 1 bell pepper, chopped (about 1 cup)
- 1 medium onion, chopped (about 1/2 cup)
- 4 ounces mushrooms, sliced (about 1 cup)
- 1 garlic clove, minced
- 1/4 teaspoon red pepper flakes
- 8 eggs
- 3 cups skim milk
- 5 cups whole-grain bakery-style bread, crusts removed and cubed
- 2/3 cup shredded low-fat pepper Jack or Cheddar cheese
- We used Chef Meg's recipe for low-sodium sausage, but the dish will work with store-bought pork, turkey or even vegetarian sausage. You could also use bacon or turkey bacon.

- Use a dense bakery-style bread rather than soft sandwich bread in this recipe. If you prefer the added texture, you can leave the crusts on the bread.5 slice Bread, mixed-grain (includes whole-grain, 7-grain)

Instructions

1. Preheat the oven to 350 degrees F if you're making this in the morning rather than the night before.
2. Coat a 9"x13" baking dish with nonstick cooking spray.
3. Cook the sausage in a nonstick skillet over medium heat. Break up the meat into bite-size chunks as it cooks. When the meat is about halfway cooked, add the pepper and onions. Cook for three minutes, until the vegetables start to soften, then add the mushrooms and garlic. Cook another two minutes, until the mushrooms have started to brown. Add the red pepper flakes and remove from heat.
4. Transfer the veggies and meat to a medium bowl to speed up the cooling process.
5. While the meat and veggies are cooling, combine eggs with milk in a medium mixing bowl.

6. Layer three cups of the bread in the bottom of the baking dish. Spoon the veggies and sausage over the bread, then sprinkle on half the cheese.
7. Carefully pour the eggs and milk into the dish, then top with the remaining bread cubes and cheese.
8. Use the back of a serving spoon to press down on the layers to help the bread soak up the eggs.
9. Cover the dish and refrigerate for up to 24 hours.
10. When you're ready to bake the dish, preheat the oven to 350 degrees.
11. Bake the casserole 35-40 minutes, until the eggs are no longer runny and the bread is golden brown.
12. Serving Size: Makes 8 servings

4. Low-Sodium Sausage

Prep Time: 5 Minutes

Cook Time: 10 Minutes

Servings: 4

Ingredients

- 8 ounces lean (80% lean/20% fat) fresh ground pork
- 2 tablespoons chicken or vegetable Stock or apple juice
- 1/2 teaspoon thyme, dried
- 1/4 teaspoon sage, dried
- 1/2 teaspoon black pepper
- 1/2 teaspoon red pepper flakes

Instructions

1. Using your hands, thoroughly combine all ingredients in a mixing bowl. Fold a 12" sheet of waxed paper in half. Divide the sausage mixture into eight equal portions (about one tablespoon each.) and roll into balls using your hands. Place the balls on one side of the waxed paper, fold the other side over, and press to flatten the sausage into patties.

2. Coat a nonstick skillet with cooking spray. Cook the sausage over medium-high heat for 10 minutes, turning halfway. Sausage should cook until the internal temperature reaches 160 degrees Fahrenheit.

3. Makes 4 servings, two patties per serving

5. Spaghetti Squash

Prep Time: 10 Minutes

Cook Time: 25 Minutes

Servings: 6

Ingredients

- 1 spaghetti squash, cut length wise
- 2 tbsp vegetable oil
- 1 1/2 cups chopped tomato
- 1 onion, chopped
- 1 clove garlic, minced
- 3 tbsp sliced black olives
- 2 tbsp fresh chopped basil
- 3/4 cup feta cheese

Instructions

1. Preheat oven to 350 degrees F. Lightly grease a baking sheet, or line with foil.
2. Place squash face down on baking sheet, and bake for 25-35 minutes, or until sharp knife can be inserted with

little resistance. Remove squash from oven and cool enough to handle.

3. Meanwhile, heat oil in skillet over medium heat. Saute onion in oil until tender. Add garlic and saute for about 3 minutes. Stir in tomatoes and heat until warm.

4. Using a spoon or fork, scoop stringy squash meat and place in a medium bowl. Toss with sauted vegetables, basil, olives, and feta. Serve warm.

6. Minestrone Soup

Prep Time: 15 Minutes

Cook Time: 45 Minutes

Servings: 8

Ingredients

- 2 tablespoons olive oil
- 1/2 cup minced white onions (about 1 small onion)
- 1/4 cup chopped zucchini
- 1/4 cup frozen cut Italian green beans
- 1/4 cup minced celery (about 1/2 stalk)
- 2 teaspoons minced garlic (about 2 cloves)
- 4 cups vegetable broth
- 1 (15 ounce) can red kidney beans, drained
- 1 (15 ounce) can small white beans or great northern beans, drained
- 1 /2 (14 ounce) can diced tomatoes
- 1/2 cup carrots, julienned or shredded
- 2 tablespoons minced fresh parsley
- 1 teaspoons dried oregano
- 1 teaspoon salt
- 1/2 teaspoon ground black pepper

- 1/2 teaspoon dried basil
- 1/4 teaspoon dried thyme
- 1 1/2 cups hot water
- 3 cups fresh baby spinach
- 1/3 cup small shell pasta

Instructions

1. Heat two tablespoons of olive oil over medium heat in a large soup pot.
2. Saute onion, celery, garlic, green beans, and zucchini in the oil for 5 minutes or until onions begin to turn translucent.
3. Add vegetable broth to pot, plus drained tomatoes, beans, carrot, hot water, and spices.
4. Bring soup to a boil, then reduce heat and allow to simmer for 20 minutes.
5. Add spinach leaves and pasta and cook for an additional 20 minutes or until desired consistency.
6. Makes about eight 1 1/2 cup servings.

7. Roasted Parmesan Potatoes

Prep Time: 15 Minutes

Cook Time: 25 Minutes

Servings: 4

Ingredients

- 4 medium Russet Potatoes, washed skin on diced
- 1 Tbsp. olive oil
- 3 Tbsp. grated parmesan cheese
- 2 tsp. dried parsley
- 1 tsp. paprika
- 1/2 tsp. garlic powder
- 1 tsp. salt
- 1/8 tsp. cayenne pepper

Instructions

1. Preheat oven 450 degrees. Spary sheet pan with cooking spray. Slice potatoes in half then cut into half inch cubes. Place potatoes in a medium bowl and toss with oil. Combine parmesan, parsley, paprika, garlic powder, salt, and cayenne pepper in a small bowl. Add

Parmesan mixture to potatoes. Toss to coat evenly. Arrange Potatoes on baking sheet. Bake, turing once until potatoes are lightly browned and easily pierced with a knife, about 25 min.

8. Slow Cooker Chicken Tortilla Soup

Prep Time: 30 Minutes

Cook Time: 4hrs 2 Minutes

Servings: 8

Ingredients

- 1 pound frozen chicken (shred near end of cooking time)
- 1 (15 ounce) can whole peeled tomatoes, mashed
- 1 (10 ounce) can enchilada sauce
- 1 medium onion, chopped
- 1 (4 ounce) can chopped green chile peppers
- 2 cloves garlic, minced
- 3(14.5 ounce) cans chicken broth
- 1 teaspoon cumin
- 1/4 teaspoon black pepper
- 1 (10 ounce) package frozen corn
- 1 can black beans, rinsed

Instructions

2. Place chicken, tomatoes, enchilada sauce, onion, green chiles, and garlic into a slow cooker. Pour in chicken broth, and season with cumin, salt, and pepper. Stir in corn and black beans. Cover and cook on Low setting for 6 to 8 hours or on High setting for 3 to 4 hours. Garnish with crushed tortilla chips, sour cream, shredded cheese, or avocados. Makes 8 servings.

9. Self-Crust Pumpkin Pie

Prep Time: 5 Minutes

Cook Time: 5 Minutes

Servings: 8

Ingredients

- 1/2 c. fat free egg substitute
- 15 oz can pure pumpkin
- 1/3 c. white sugar
- 1/3 c. packed brown sugar
- 1/4 tsp. salt
- 1 1/2 tsp cinnamon
- 3 tbsp white flour
- 1 c. dry milk
- 1 c. water

Instructions

1. Mix all ingredients except water together
3. In a large bowl.
2. Gradually stir in water until well mixed.
3. Spray a 9-inch pan with cooking spray.

4. Pour batter into pan.

5. Bake at 350Â° for 45-55 minutes

6. Or until knife inserted 1 inch from the center

7. Comes out clean.

8. Keep pie chilled after cooking.

10. Parmesan Herb Baked Tilapia

Prep Time: 30 Minutes

Cook Time: 10 Minutes

Servings: 4

Ingredients

- 4 (6-oz) tilapia fillets
- Cooking spray
- 1/3 cup grated parmesan cheese
- 1/4 cup fat free mayonnaise
- 2 T minced green onions
- 1/4 cup dry breadcrumbs
- 1 tsp dried basil
- 1 tsp dried oregano
- 1/4 tsp salt
- 1/4 tsp black pepper

Instructions

1. Preheat oven to 400 degrees. Place fish on a foil-lined baking sheet coated with cooking spray. Combine cheese, mayonnaise, and onions; spread evenly over

fish. Combine breadcrumbs and remaining ingredients; sprinkle evenly over fish. Lightly coat fish with cooking spray. Bake at 400 degrees for 10 minutes or until fish flakes easily when tested with a fork. Makes 4 servings

LUNCH

11. Slow Cooker BBQ Pulled Pork Roast

Prep Time: 10 Minutes

Cook Time: 3hrs 2 Minutes

Servings: 12

Ingredients

- 1 cup chopped celery
- 1 cup chopped onions
- 1 cup ketchup
- 1 cup barbecue sauce
- 1 cup water
- 2 tbsp vinegar
- 2 tbsp Worcestershire sauce
- 2 tbsp brown sugar
- 1 tsp chili powder
- 1 tsp salt
- 1/2 tsp pepper
- 1/2 tsp garlic powder
- 3 lbs boneless pork roast

Instructions

2. Combine all ingredients except roast in the slow cooker.
3. Add the roast.
4. Cover, cook on high for 6-7 hours.
5. Remove the roast.
6. Shred the meat, and return it to the sauce.
7. If desired, thicken the sauce by simmering on the stovetop.
8. Great for making sandwiches or using in other recipes. The sauce is good on rice, too.

12. Guilt Free Pineapple Orange Cake

Prep Time: 15 Minutes

Cook Time: 25 Minutes

Servings: 15

Ingredients

- 1 package yellow cake mix
- 1 can (11 oz) mandarin oranges, undrained
- 4 egg whites
- 1/2 cup unsweetened applesauce

Topping:

- 1 can (20 oz) crushed pineapple, undrained
- 1 package sugar-free instant vanilla pudding mix
- 1 carton (8oz) reduced-fat whipped topping

Instructions

1. In a large mixing bowl, beat the cake mix, oranges, and egg whites and applesauce on low speed for 2 minutes. Pour into a 13-in x 9 in baking dish coated with nonstick cooking spray.

2. Bake at 350 degrees for 25-30 minutes or until a toothpick inserted near the center comes out clean. Cool on a wire rack.

3. In a bowl, combine the pineapple and pudding mix. Fold in whipped topping just until blended. Spread over cake. Refrigerate for at least 1 hour before serving.

4. Makes 15 servings.

13. Spicy Taco Soup

Prep Time: 5 Minutes

Cook Time: 20 Minutes

Servings: 8

Ingredients

- 1 lb ground beef
- 1 onion, chopped
- 2 (14.5 oz) cans diced tomatoes with green chilies
- 2 (14.5 oz) cans pinto beans (drained)
- 1 (14.5 oz) can black beans (drained)
- 1 (14.5 oz) can cream-style corn
- 1 package ranch style dressing mix
- 1 package taco seasoning
- 1 cup water (or broth) optional

Instructions

1. Brown beef with onions in a medium soup pot. Drain excess grease. Add remaining ingredients, stir and simmer for 20 minutes. If it seems a little thick you can add some beef broth or water.

2. This is great with cilantro and a dab of sour cream!

3. 8 servings of about 1 1/2 cups each

14. Rustic Italian Tortellini Soup

Prep Time: 10 Minutes

Cook Time: 20 Minutes

Servings: 6

Ingredients

- 3 Italian turkey sausage links (4 ounces each), casings removed (I used the "hot" sausage version)
- 1 medium onion, chopped
- 6 garlic cloves, minced
- 4 cups reduced-sodium chicken broth
- 1 can (14-1/2 ounces) diced tomatoes, undrained
- 1 package (9 ounces) refrigerated cheese tortellini
- 1 package (6 ounces) fresh baby spinach, coarsely chopped
- 2-1/4 teaspoons minced fresh basil or 3/4 teaspoon dried basil (or, you can substitute thyme and oregano)
- 1/4 teaspoon pepper
- Dash crushed red pepper flakes (optional if not using hot turkey sausage)
- Shredded Parmesan cheese, optional

Instructions

1. Crumble sausage into a Dutch oven; add onion. Cook and stir over medium heat until meat is no longer pink.
2. Add garlic; cook and stir 2 minutes longer.
3. Add the broth and tomatoes. Bring to a boil.
4. Stir in tortellini; return to a boil. Reduce heat; simmer, uncovered, for 5-8 minutes or until pasta is tender, stirring occasionally.
5. Add the spinach, basil, pepper and pepper flakes; cook 2-3 minutes longer or until spinach is wilted. Serve with cheese if desired.
6. Yield: 6 servings (2 quarts

15. Broiled Tilapia Parmesan

Prep Time: 5 Minutes

Cook Time: 10 Minutes

Servings: 4

Ingredients

- 1/4 cup Parmesan cheese
- 2 tablespoons butter, softened
- 1 tablespoon and 1-1/2 teaspoons reduced-fat mayonnaise
- 1 tablespoon fresh lemon juice
- 1/8 teaspoon dried basil
- 1/8 teaspoon ground black pepper
- 1/8 teaspoon onion powder
- 1/8 teaspoon celery seed
- 1 pound tilapia fillets

Instructions

1. Preheat your oven's broiler. Grease a broiling pan or line pan with aluminum foil.

2. In a small bowl, mix together the Parmesan cheese, butter, mayonnaise and lemon juice. Season with dried basil, pepper, onion powder and celery salt. Mix well and set aside.

3. Arrange fillets in a single layer on the prepared pan. Broil a few inches from the heat for 2 to 3 minutes. Flip the fillets over and broil for a couple more minutes. Remove the fillets from the oven and cover them with the Parmesan cheese mixture on the top side. Broil for 2 more minutes or until the topping is browned and fish flakes easily with a fork. Be careful not to overcook the fish.

4. Makes 4 servings.

16. Sherry's Cucumber Salad

Prep Time: 15 Minutes

Cook Time: 00 Minutes

Servings: 4

Ingredients

- 2 large cucumbers sliced thinly,peel optional
- 1 medium tomatoes,chopped
- 1/2 medium red onion,chopped
- 1 bell pepper,chopped
- 1/4 cup Kraft Fat Free Italian dressing
- Optional Items
- Make this salad into a quick dinner or side
- Dish by using some of the following items.
- Fresh Lettuces or Salad Greens
- Whole Grain Pasta
- Fresh Mozzerella
- Hard Salami
- Genoa Salami
- Leftover rotisserie Chicken

Instructions

1. In a large bowl add the sliced cucumber, chopped tomato, chopped onion, chopped bell pepper.Add salad dressing to the bowl.It may not look like enough dressing, but the veggies will add more moisture.Stir the salad, and refrigerate for 1 hour stirring after 30 minutes.Serve and enjoy.

Options:

2. 1 Serve on a bed of fresh lettuce or salad greens
3. 2 Serve as a side dish by stirring in 2 cups of
4. Cooked whole grain pasta
5. 3 Add 1/2 cup of fresh mozzerella,chopped and
6. 1/2 cup of diced hard,or Genoa salamibefore

Marinating

1. 4 Add 1 cup of chopped,leftover rotisserie
2. Chicken and serve over salad greens

17. Easy Ground Beef Skillet

Prep Time: 5 Minutes

Cook Time: 25 Minutes

Servings: 4

Ingredients

- 1 tsp olive oil
- 1/4 cup chopped onion
- 1 lg clove garlic (pressed or minced)
- 1 lb 96% lean ground beef
- 2 tbsp flour
- 1 c 2% milk
- 1/2 tsp ground cumin
- 1/2 tsp ground sage
- 1/4 tsp salt
- 12 oz bag frozen mixed veggies (corn, carrots, green beans, etc)

Instructions

1. Heat olive oil in large skillet (10"-12") over medium heat.

2. Add onion and cook until browned.

3. Add garlic.

4. Add ground beef and cook until browned.

5. Sprinkle flour evenly over mixture in pan and stir well.

6. Add milk in small amounts, stirring well each time.

7. Add cumin, sage and salt.

8. Add frozen veggies and continue to cook for a few more minutes (or until desired tenderness).

9. Makes 4 - 1 cup (approx) servings

10. Variations: Try using different spices to adjust to your taste or try different mixes of veggies

18. Low-Fat, Whole-Wheat, Fresh Strawberry and Dark Chocolate Scones

Prep Time: 10 Minutes

Cook Time: 15 Minutes

Servings: 8

Ingredients

- 1.5 Cup whole wheat Pastry flour
- .5 Cup Whole Wheat Flour
- .25 Cup Oat Bran
- 1 tbsp Baking Powder
- 3 Tbsp turbinado sugar
- 1/8 tsp Salt
- 5 Tbsp cold, unsalted butter
- 1 cup chopped fresh strawberries
- 4 squares of ghiradellli 60% Cocao Chocolate Bar
- .5 cup almond milk (or any milk on hand)
- .5 cup Greek Yogurt (I used Chobani plain, non-fat)
- 1 tsp Vanilla extract

Instructions

1. Pre-heat oven to 425 degrees F. Put Parchment paper on a baking sheet.
2. Whisk the first 5 ingredients together until blended.
3. Cut the cold butter into smaller pieces and cut it into the flour. You could also use a food processor to speed this step up a bit
4. Chop the squares of chocolate into smaller pieces and add the chocolate and strawberries to the flour and butter mixture until they a evenly coated.
5. Pour in the almond milk and greek yogurt to the bowl. Stir until mostly combined, use your hands to mix well.
6. Take the dough and set it on your prepared baking pan. Form it into a flat circle and cut it into 8 triangles.
7. Space the scones out on the baking pan, and bake for 15-20 minutes, until lightly browned and firm.

19. Skillet Lasagna

Prep Time: 10 Minutes

Cook Time: 20 Minutes

Servings: 6

Ingredients

- 1 pound lean ground beef
- 1 small onion (chopped)
- 3 cloves garlic (minced)
- 1 (14-ounce) can diced tomatoes (undrained)
- 1 1/4 cups water
- 8 ounces tomato sauce
- 1 tbsp dried parsley flakes
- 1 tsp dried basil leaves
- 1 tsp dried oregano leaves
- 1 tsp salt
- 2 1/2 cups broken-up whole wheat lasagna noodles
- 1 cup fat-free cottage cheese
- 1/4 cup fat-free grated Parmesan cheese
- Dash dried basil and pepper (optional)
- 1 egg
- Shredded fat-free mozzarella cheese for garnish

Instructions

1. In a large skillet, brown beef with onions and garlic. Drain.
2. Add tomatoes, water, tomato sauce, parsley, basil, oregano, and salt.
3. Stir in uncooked pasta.
4. Bring to a boil, stirring occasionally.
5. Reduce heat, cover and simmer for 20 minutes or until pasta is tender.
6. Combine cottage and Parmesan cheeses.
7. Mix in the egg.
8. Sprinkle in basil and pepper to taste.
9. Drop cheese mixture by rounded tablespoons onto pasta mixture.
10. Cover and cook for 5 minutes more.
11. Sprinkle with shredded mozzarella and serve.

20. Garlic Brown Sugar Chicken

Prep Time: 5 Minutes

Cook Time: 15 Minutes

Servings: 4

Ingredients

- 4 tsp brown sugar
- 12 ounces boneless, skinless chicken breasts
- 1 clove garlic
- 2 Tbsp butter
- Dash black pepper

Instructions

1. This makes four servings, 3 oz per person
2. Melt the butter in a frying pan.
3. Brown the garlic in the butter.
4. Add chicken breasts to garlic and butter and cook thoroughly, adding pepper as you like it.
5. When chicken is fully cooked add brown sugar on top of each breast.

6. Allow the brown sugar to melt into the chicken (about 5 minutes).

7. Serve with your favorite carb, and veggie or salad. We usually have rice or noodles and carrots or green beans.

DINNER

21. Sesame Brown Rice Salad with Shredded Chicken and Peanuts

Prep Time: 5 Minutes

Cook Time: 15 Minutes

Servings: 4

Ingredients

- 1 cup long-grain brown rice
- 2 cups shredded cooked chicken breast
- ½ cup shredded carrot
- ⅓ Cup sliced green onions
- ¼ cup dry-roasted peanuts, divided
- 1 tablespoon chopped fresh cilantro, divided
- ½ teaspoon salt
- 2 tablespoons fresh lime juice
- 4 teaspoons canola oil
- 1 teaspoon dark sesame oil
- 2 garlic cloves, minced

Instruction

1. Cook rice according to package directions, omitting salt and fat. Transfer rice to a large bowl; fluff with a fork. Cool. Add chicken, carrot, onions, 2 tablespoons peanuts, 2 teaspoons cilantro, and salt to rice; toss to combine.

2. Combine juice and remaining ingredients in a small bowl. Drizzle oil mixture over rice mixture; toss to combine. Place 1 1/2 cups salad on each of 4 plates. Sprinkle each serving with 1 1/2 teaspoons remaining peanuts and 1/4 teaspoon remaining cilantro.

22. Cider-Glazed Chicken with Browned Butter-Pecan Rice

Prep Time: 5 Minutes

Cook Time: 15 Minutes

Servings: 4

Ingredients

- 1 (3.5-ounce) bag boil-in-bag brown rice (such as Uncle Ben's)
- 2 tablespoons butter, divided
- 1 pound chicken breast cutlets (about 4 cutlets)
- ¾ teaspoon salt, divided
- ¼ teaspoon freshly ground black pepper
- ½ cup refrigerated apple cider
- 1 teaspoon Dijon mustard
- ¼ cup chopped pecans
- 2 tablespoons chopped fresh flat-leaf parsley

Instructions

1. Cook rice according to package directions in a small saucepan, omitting salt and fat; drain.

2. While rice cooks, melt 1 teaspoon butter in a large heavy skillet over medium-high heat. Sprinkle chicken with 1/4 teaspoon salt and pepper. Add chicken to pan; cook 3 minutes on each side or until done. Remove from pan. Add cider and mustard to pan, scraping pan to loosen browned bits; cook 2 to 3 minutes or until syrupy. Add chicken to pan, turning to coat. Remove from heat; set aside.

3. Melt remaining 5 teaspoons butter in saucepan over medium-high heat; cook for 2 minutes or until browned and fragrant. Lower heat to medium; add pecans, and cook for 1 minute or until toasted, stirring frequently. Add rice and the remaining 1/2 teaspoon salt; toss well to coat. Serve rice with chicken. Sprinkle with parsley.

23. Chicken, Broccoli, and Brown Rice Casserole

Prep Time: 10 Minutes

Cook Time: 20 Minutes

Servings: 4

Ingredients

- 2 (3 1/2-ounce) bags boil-in-bag brown rice
- 1 tablespoon olive oil
- 1 small onion, finely chopped (about 1 cup)
- 8 ounces presliced button mushrooms
- 8 ounces skinless, boneless chicken thighs, cut into bite-sized pieces
- ¾ teaspoon salt, divided
- ¼ teaspoon freshly ground black pepper
- 1 (12-ounce) bag microwave-in-bag fresh broccoli florets
- 1 ½ cups 1% low-fat milk
- 3 tablespoons all-purpose flour
- 3 ounces sharp cheddar cheese, shredded (about 3/4 cup)

Instructions

1. Preheat broiler to high. Cook rice according to package directions; drain.
2. While rice cooks, heat a large 12-inch ovenproof skillet over medium-high heat. Add oil to pan; swirl to coat. Add onion, mushrooms, and chicken; sprinkle with 1/4 teaspoon salt and pepper. Sauté 6 minutes or until chicken and onion are d
3. Cook broccoli in microwave according to package directions for 3 minutes. Open package to release steam
4. Combine milk and flour, stirring with a whisk or fork until smoo
5. Stir milk mixture into chicken mixture in skille
6. Cook 2 minutes or until bubbly and thick, stirring frequent
7. Stir in remaining 1/2 teaspoon salt, rice, and broccoli. Sprinkle with cheese.
8. Broil 1 minute or until cheese melts and just begins to brown
9. Riff: Try ground beef in place of the chicken.
10. Riff: Not a fan of broccoli? Try cauliflower, spinach, green peas, carrots, or green beans instead.

11. Riff: In place of rice, use 3 cups cooked quinoa (1 cup
    uncooked).

24. Spicy Peanut Chicken over Rice

Prep Time: 10 Minutes

Cook Time: 30 Minutes

Servings: 12

Ingredients

- 1 tablespoon peanut oil
- 1 cup chopped onion (about 1 medium)
- 1 ½ tablespoons minced garlic (about 4 cloves)
- 2 ½ pounds skinless, boneless chicken breast halves, cut into 1-inch pieces
- ⅓ Cup chunky peanut butter
- 1 ½ teaspoons curry powder
- 1 teaspoon salt
- 1 teaspoon crushed red pepper
- ½ teaspoon freshly ground black pepper
- 1 (6-ounce) can tomato paste
- 3 cups chopped plum tomato (about 6 tomatoes)
- 2 (14-ounce) cans fat-free, less-sodium chicken broth
- 8 cups hot cooked brown rice
- ¾ cup 2% Greek-style yogurt (such as Fage)

Instructions

1. Heat oil in a Dutch oven over medium heat. Add onion and garlic to pan; cook 5 minutes or until tender, stirring frequently. Add chicken to pan; cook 4 minutes or until chicken is done, stirring frequently. Stir in peanut butter and next 5 ingredients (through tomato paste); cook 1 minute. Add tomato and broth to pan; bring to a boil. Reduce heat, and simmer 30 minutes or until slightly thickened, stirring occasionally. Serve chicken mixture over rice; top each serving with yogurt.

25. Middle Eastern Rice Salad

Prep Time: 15 Minutes

Cook Time: 5 Minutes

Servings: 4

Ingredients

- 2 tablespoons olive oil
- ½ Vidalia or other sweet onion, thinly sliced (about 3/4 cup)
- 1 (16-ounce) can chickpeas, rinsed and drained
- ½ teaspoon ground cumin
- ¼ teaspoon salt
- Freshly ground black pepper
- 3 cups cooked brown rice
- ½ cup chopped pitted dates
- ¼ cup chopped fresh mint
- ¼ cup chopped fresh parsley

Instructions

2. Heat oil in a large nonstick skillet over medium-high heat. Add onion, and cook, stirring often, about 5

minutes or until onion begins to brown. Remove from heat, and stir in chickpeas, cumin, and salt. Season to taste with freshly ground black pepper.

3. Combine rice, onion-chickpea mixture, dates, mint, and parsley in a large bowl. Toss well until thoroughly combined. Serve warm or at room temperature.

26. Summer Veggie Rice Bowl

Prep Time: 12 Minutes

Cook Time: 1hr 3 Minutes

Servings: 4

Ingredients

- 1 ⅓ cups cooked brown rice, cooled to room temperature
- 1 cup frozen shelled edamame (green soybeans), thawed
- 1 cup grape tomatoes, halved
- ½ cup torn fresh basil
- ¼ cup pine nuts, toasted
- 2 teaspoons grated lemon rind
- 3 tablespoons fresh lemon juice
- 1 teaspoon kosher salt
- ¼ teaspoon freshly ground black pepper
- 3 tablespoons olive oil, divided
- 2 cups chopped zucchini
- ½ ounce fresh Parmesan cheese, shaved

Instructions

1. Combine the first 9 ingredients in a large bowl, and toss until well blended. Heat a medium skillet over medium-high heat. Add 1 tablespoon olive oil to pan; swirl to coat. Add zucchini; sauté 4 minutes, stirring occasionally. Add zucchini and remaining 2 tablespoons oil to rice mixture; toss. Top with shaved Parmesan cheese.

27. Hummus-and-Rice Fritters with Mediterranean Salad

Prep Time: 25 Minutes

Cook Time: 00 Minutes

Servings: 4

Ingredients

- 1 ½ cups precooked packaged brown rice (such as Uncle Ben's)
- 1 cup prepared traditional hummus (such as Sabra Classic Hummus)
- 3 tablespoons cake flour
- ⅛ Teaspoon ground red pepper
- 1 large egg white
- 7 teaspoons extra-virgin olive oil, divided
- ½ teaspoon kosher salt, divided
- 1 tablespoon fresh lemon juice
- ¼ teaspoon freshly ground black pepper
- 2 cups baby arugula
- 1 cup halved cherry tomatoes
- 1 cup diagonally cut slices seeded peeled cucumber
- ½ cup thinly sliced red onion
- 1 ounce goat cheese, crumbled (about 1/4 cup)

Instructions

1. Place first 5 ingredients in a food processor; process until smooth. Heat a large nonstick skillet over medium heat. Add 2 teaspoons oil to pan; swirl to coat. Add 4 (1/4-cup) batter mounds to pan, pressing each with the back of a spatula to flatten slightly. Cook 4 minutes on each side or until golden and thoroughly cooked. Remove from pan; keep warm. Repeat procedure with 2 teaspoons oil and remaining batter. Sprinkle fritters with 1/4 teaspoon salt.

2. Combine remaining 1 tablespoon oil, remaining 1/4 teaspoon salt, lemon juice, and black pepper in a large bowl, stirring with a whisk. Add arugula, cherry tomatoes, cucumber, and onion; toss gently to coat. Arrange about 1 cup salad, 2 fritters, and 1 tablespoon goat cheese on each of 4 plates. Serve immediately.

28. Slow Cooker Sweet-and-Sour Chicken

Prep Time: 25 Minutes

Cook Time: 8hrs 2 Minutes

Servings: 6

Ingredients

- 1 ¼ pounds boneless, skinless chicken thighs
- 2 cups chopped red bell pepper
- 1 ½ cups unsalted chicken stock
- 1 cup chopped yellow onion
- 1 cup thinly sliced carrots
- ¼ cup lower-sodium soy sauce
- 2 tablespoons lower-sodium Worcestershire sauce
- 1 tablespoon sambal oelek (ground fresh chile paste)
- ¾ cup unsalted ketchup, divided
- ¼ cup pineapple juice
- 2 tablespoons cornstarch
- 3 cups cooked brown rice
- 1 ½ teaspoons sesame seeds
- 1 ½ teaspoons sliced scallions

Instructions

1. Add chicken, bell pepper, chicken stock, onion, carrots, soy sauce, Worcestershire sauce, sambal oelek, and 1/2 cup ketchup to a 6-quart slow cooker. Cover and cook on low until chicken shreds easily with a fork, about 7 hours. Remove chicken from slow cooker. Shred chicken, and cover to keep warm.

2. Whisk together pineapple juice and cornstarch in a small bowl. Increase slow cooker heat to high; slowly stir in pineapple juice mixture and remaining 1/4 cup ketchup. Cook, uncovered, until sauce is thick enough to coat the back of a spoon, about 30 minutes. Stir in chicken. Serve over rice, and sprinkle with sesame seeds and scallions.

29. Lemon Chicken Teriyaki Rice Bowl

Prep Time: 28 Minutes

Cook Time: 20 Minutes

Servings: 4

Ingredients

- 1 cup long-grain brown rice
- 2 tablespoons lower-sodium soy sauce
- ½ teaspoon cornstarch
- 2 tablespoons dark brown sugar
- 4 teaspoons mirin (sweet rice wine)
- 2 teaspoons fresh lemon juice
- 3 (6-ounce) skinless, boneless chicken breast halves
- ¼ teaspoon kosher salt
- ¼ teaspoon black pepper
- 2 teaspoons canola oil
- 1 pound Broccolini, trimmed

Instructions

1. Preheat oven to 400°. Cook brown rice according to directions. Combine soy sauce and cornstarch in a

small saucepan, stirring with a whisk. Add brown sugar, mirin, and lemon juice; bring to a boil. Cook 1 minute or until thickened. Sprinkle chicken with salt and pepper. Heat a large ovenproof skillet over medium-high heat. Add canola oil to pan; swirl to coat. Add chicken to pan; cook 4 minutes. Turn; drizzle 1 tablespoon soy sauce mixture over chicken. Place pan in oven; bake at 400° for 8 minutes or until done. Place chicken on a cutting board; let stand 5 minutes. Cut chicken into slices. Bring a large saucepan of water to a boil. Add Broccolini; cook 3 minutes or until crisp-tender. Drain. Place 1/2 cup rice in each of 4 bowls; top each serving with 4 ounces chicken and 4 ounces Broccolini. Drizzle about 1 tablespoon remaining soy sauce mixture over each serving.

30. Chicken and Rice Noodle Stir-Fry with Ginger and Basil

Prep Time: 18 Minutes

Cook Time: 00 Minutes

Servings: 4

Ingredients

- 4 ounces uncooked brown rice noodles
- ¼ cup unsalted chicken stock
- 2 tablespoons oyster sauce
- 1 tablespoon lower-sodium soy sauce
- 2 teaspoons rice vinegar
- 1 teaspoon sambal oelek
- 1 tablespoon canola oil
- 1 pound skinless, boneless chicken breast halves, cut into 1/4-inch-thick slices
- 1 tablespoon canola oil
- 6 ounces shiitake mushrooms, sliced
- 1 ½ tablespoons minced peeled fresh ginger
- 1 red bell pepper, thinly sliced
- 1 tablespoon minced garlic
- 4 green onions, sliced
- ⅔ Cup torn fresh basil leaves

Instructions

2. Prepare noodles according to package directions. Drain; rinse with cold water. Drain. Combine chicken stock, oyster sauce, soy sauce, vinegar, and sambal oelek in a bowl. Heat a large wok or skillet over high heat. Add 1 tablespoon canola oil; swirl. Add chicken to pan; cook 1 1/2 minutes on each side. Remove chicken from pan. Add 1 tablespoon canola oil to pan; swirl. Add mushrooms; stir-fry 1 minute. Add ginger and sliced bell pepper; stir-fry 1 minute. Add minced garlic and sliced green onions; stir-fry 30 seconds. Add noodles, stock mixture, and chicken; cook 1 minute. Stir in basil.